In a world both beautiful and painful,
in which we have some—but not total—control,
my regular practice of reflection
and micro-commitments to be My Better Self
help me not just survive but thrive and
be more grateful for each day and
more committed to finding happiness and compassion.

As you join the Monday Minutes conversation,
I hope you find those things, too.

The 52 messages and journaling opportunities
invite you to take a few minutes each week
to think about memories that matter
or make a little goal (or a big one)
and move toward Your Better Self, too.

You can journal in order by page or skip around
to topics that speak to you in the moment.
Date your entries, if you like.
This record of who you are, and have been, and want to be
is a gift to you from yourself
and (should you choose) for future generations.
You matter, now and to the future.

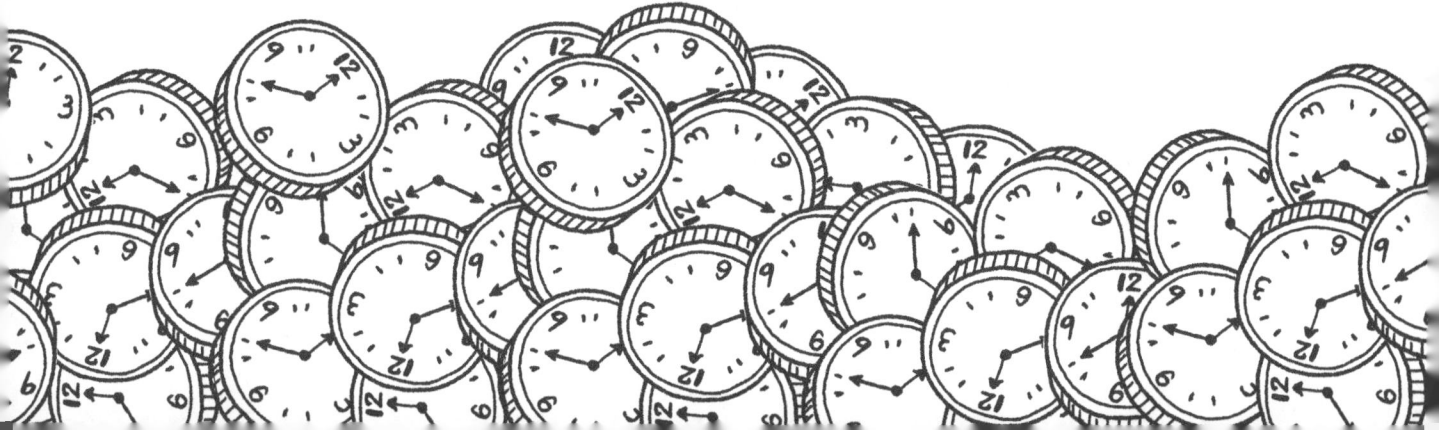

Layout and icon design by Carrie Svozil.

Printed in the United States of America

ISBN 978-1-7346139-5-7 Print
ISBN 978-1-7346139-6-4 eBook

Your DNA Guide
info@yourDNAguide.com
www.yourDNAguide.com

Acknowledgments

I want to thank Sunny Morton for her careful, thoughtful, and articulate editing skills for the Monday Minutes series. She takes my sometimes rambling, nonsensical thoughts and makes them more coherent, concise, and powerful. This series simply would not be what it is without her talent and insight. Plus, it was her idea to make our Monday Minutes book into a journal, which I am just thrilled about.

I also want to thank Kathie Knoll for her initial brainchild to put Monday Minutes into print, and her efforts to take an overwhelming amount of content and whittle it down to just 52 entries that offer a balance of humor and gravity, of past and future ideas. And also for just being my best cheerleader.

Why semi trucks have so many mirrors

Did you know that semi trucks have at least two sets of mirrors? One up at their own eye level and one down at the regular traffic level. Some trucks have mirrors on the front corners of the hood, too. That's a lot of mirrors.

I asked someone who drives a big bus why they need so many. He said that while the big mirrors up by the driver do provide a great view of most of the road, they actually don't show what's immediately next to them! Such as me, in my much-littler car.

It made me think about how I am looking around and behind myself, metaphorically speaking. (At the beginning of the new year, I have thoughts like this.) Too often, I am using only my rearview mirrors and only for selective hindsight: to look back and notice only the lack in myself and only the success of others.

But if I actually look ALL around myself, I will be more aware of others alongside me. I will move forward more confidently and safely. I can be inspired (or warned) by their driving. I may even notice spots on the road where a car just my size would fit even better.

Now I'm finding more value in that full, 360-degree perspective. It helps me decide if and when I should change lanes, or stay where I am.

What will you do this year? Will you be changing lanes or staying the course? I hope you glance in lots of mirrors–not just the rearview mirror–to help you make great decisions on your road ahead.

How do you check different angles before making a decision?

Write about a time when you needed more than one perspective to understand a situation.

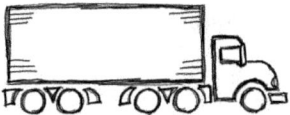

Just pave over your obstacles already

There is a Costco just down the street from my house. Like many Costco stores, the entrance is triangular, with the parking lot on three sides of the building.

They recently redid the sidewalk and parking lot area directly in front of the entrance. I think they paved over a flower bed because people were walking through it. It was, after all, the most direct route to the entrance.

How many years did it take for Costco to decide to pull out the flower bed? How many years before someone stopped hoping people would change and walk around it? Did someone trip on a bush, so their lawyer finally told them it had to go?

This made me think about the things in my life that are keeping me from getting directly where I want to go. How many years have I been going around or trudging through some obstacles when I should just rip them out and pave the way?

I hope your route is sensibly smooth and that you are getting where you want to go. If you will excuse me, I have some ripping out and removal to do.

Reflect on a time when you overcame a challenge by changing your approach.

How can you make your path smoother this week?

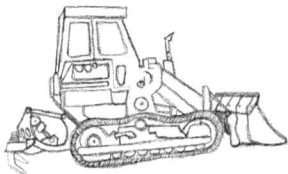

Stopped, with no train in sight

I recently found myself stopped at the train tracks before those white and red striped crossing barriers, waiting for the train to appear. Slowly cars began to pile up behind me.

A full minute went by. No train. I could see the driver on the other side straining to see further down the track, and I was doing the same. Granted, I couldn't see too far down the tracks, but I definitely did not see a train. What to do? How long do I sit here and wait? Am I even brave enough to break the law and cross a train track while the barriers are down?

Well, the guy across the road from me skirted around the guards and began to cross the tracks. My mind immediately conjured up a gruesome scene of a train crashing through his car and derailing. But that didn't happen. The car successfully navigated the guard rails and sped off down the road.

It made me wonder about that balance between patience (or prudence) and action. Certainly, there is a time for each, but how do we know when to do what? How do we know when it is action that will bring the best outcome, or just enduring?

I don't know the answer. But I do know that soon after that car went around the barrier, the gates raised back up and I drove through the intersection, never having encountered a train. I realized that inaction is an action. It is still a choice. So if I am sitting still, it better be because I am choosing to, not just because I am afraid to move forward.

Do you tend more toward patience or action? Do you want to change?

Reflect on a time you had to decide between patience and action. How did it turn out?

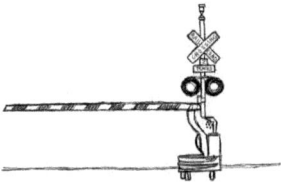

Slippery sidewalks and assumptions

I have a love/hate relationship with my neighborhood's homeowner's association (HOA). I love the overall beauty of our neighborhood, which they support. In the spring when they threaten me with fines for unpulled weeds in the rocks by my garage, I don't love them.

Recently, my husband and I were out walking after a snowstorm. After a snowy section of sidewalk, I commented, "I am surprised the HOA doesn't fine people for not shoveling their sidewalks."

He responded with a simple question: "How do you know they don't?"

I immediately understood his logic. Since we do shovel our sidewalks, I have no idea if the HOA fines those who don't.

Why was I so confident in making a statement that I literally had zero evidence to back up? I was assuming that if the HOA did impose fines, everyone would shovel their sidewalks. Clearly, that logic is flawed.

Maybe this kind of flawed logic isn't so bad when we are just thinking about slippery sidewalks. But it has made me examine my other assumptions and recognize them for what they are. What other things do I just assume without evidence? I hope I'll be more careful on those slippery assumptions...and any slippery sidewalks, too.

What is an assumption you've made that you might want to rethink?

Reflect on a time when you misjudged a situation or person.

To be or not to be...a bot

I was ordering contact lenses online the other day for my daughter, who had apparently been wearing two right-eyed contacts for the past several weeks and just kept forgetting to mention that she needed more. I filled out all the required information.

The screen began spinning. A phrase appeared: "Verifying you are human. This may take a few seconds."

I appreciated the clever attempt at humor, but I couldn't help but wonder, "How are they verifying I am human?"

Presumably, the intent was to verify what I was NOT: some computer bot, trolling the internet for information that could be used for nefarious purposes. They weren't really verifying what I was...my humanity.

"Not being a bot" is a fairly easy test to pass: I can read information on a screen and give appropriate feedback. But that is not really what makes me human.

I am sure there are scientific definitions of our species. But, to me, what makes me and you deserving of the title of "human" is that we innovate and change and adapt and feel and fail and love. We have the capacity to learn and build and create.

I hope you, like me, don't want to be defined by what you are not, but instead by what you are.

Write about a moment when you felt truly seen for who you are.

Reflect on a time you felt misunderstood.

Date

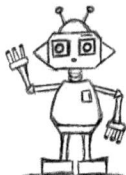

I saw this on a public bus

I was recently on an overcrowded public bus in a big city outside the United States. There were three doors on the bus, but only the front door had a payment reader. There was no way those entering in the back two doors could make it up to the front to pay. With all the people coming in and out, it seemed like it would be very easy to just not pay.

Without fail, every person who boarded in the back passed their bus pass toward the front. No one said anything about it. This was obviously just common practice, as each person passed it up to the next person and so on. A minute or so later the card came back and the passenger tucked it back into a pocket or wallet.

I was impressed first with the honesty of these passengers and then I was struck by the beauty of this social norm. It is a simple thing, to pass a bus pass up and then back, but it was done so effortlessly that it made me wish that other areas of our lives were so fully supported by each other.

This week I am going to look for everyday ways I can help those around me feel more supported in what they are trying to do. I hope you will too.

Write about a time you noticed strangers doing something good.

List several things you're grateful for in this moment.

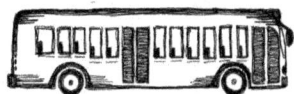

That moment in the car in my wedding dress

What do you recall about one of the best or most meaningful days of your life? For me, it was my wedding day.

Strangely enough, of all the things I remember about that day, I have thought about one specific moment many, many times in the years following.

I was by myself in the passenger seat of our red Mercury Sable, my big poofy wedding dress taking up my entire side of the car. My husband (!!) was right next to the door, with his back to me, putting gas into the car.

Why did I think of that moment so many times afterward? It helped me remember which side of the car the gas tank was on.

Yes, a very practical reason to think on that moment, but doing it with so much frequency did not diminish those feelings of joy and anticipation, and disbelief even, that I had just been married. I am grateful that those feelings are anchored in that simple moment, and that I had a practical reason to keep them with me often.

I hope you can reflect on a similar, everyday moment, and that it still carries some treasured feelings for you.

Write about a small moment you remember from a big day.

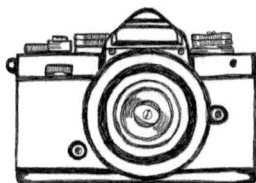

My mom put "team" in "softball team"

When my mom passed, we held a Celebration of Life open house. (I think it is SO IMPORTANT to hold some kind of something to allow people to gather and connect after a loved one passes.) I loved it. I loved seeing friends and cousins. Loved how most of them commented on our display of pictures and volunteer badges and newspaper clippings that they had learned something new about my mom.

My favorite moment was when two women I didn't recognize presented my sister and me with a picture of my mom on a softball team they had played on together in 1976 (my sister is actually in utero in the picture!). The two women expressed how grateful they were for my mom and how she made them feel welcome and accepted on the team. This was a very big deal for two lesbian women in the mid '70's.

I had never heard anything about them or this story. But I was so touched that after all these years, my mom's inclusion and kindness meant so much that they attended a gathering where they wouldn't know anyone to celebrate a woman they hadn't seen in nearly 50 years. But their experience with my mom embodies that of so many others with her. She accepted everyone.

I am going to be a little more like that this week. I hope you will too.

What is a small kindness someone has done for you that you'll always remember?

Share a story about someone you love that captures something about them.

A tender moment in a random parking lot

I was a backseat passenger in an unfamiliar car in an unfamiliar place. I found myself just staring out the window and not paying that much attention to the conversation around me. It was relatively early in the morning, but the sun was up and the day was warm. We passed gas stations and strip malls, fast food restaurants and car washes.

We passed a parking lot in front of a big box store and in the five seconds it took us to drive by I took in the most tender scene. There was a big man wearing a reflective vest, t-shirt, jeans, and heavy boots. I couldn't see his face because it was nestled down next to the cheek of a little baby. He was standing in the parking lot behind his car just swaying and rocking that baby.

I craned my neck to watch them for as long as I could. What's their story? I wondered. Were they waiting for the mom to finish shopping and then he would go to work? Or had he worked all night and was now dead on his feet, trying to soothe his sweet baby?

It was one of a million simple moments that happen in everyday lives that aren't ever recorded because they don't seem significant enough. But I felt that love and connection and tenderness, and I decided you needed to know that those things still exist in the world.

Even, or maybe especially, in random parking lots in nowhere places.

Write about a moment that reminded you of goodness in the world.

When is a time you witnessed tenderness?

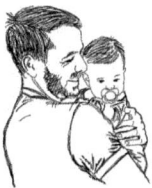

Your stories matter (Taylor Swift agrees)

I didn't expect to cry at the Taylor Swift concert.

She sang a song I had never heard called "Marjorie." In fact, I'll bet very few fans would consider this song their favorite and yet Taylor included it in her already crowded set list. The inclusion of this song made me love Taylor even more.

Majorie is a tribute to the impact Taylor's maternal grandmother had on her. Her plea to her grandma in her song is one we all need to hear: "I should've asked you questions, I should've asked you how to be, Asked you to write it down for me."

If you are the grandma (or grandpa) please know that your stories matter, but those they matter to often don't realize how much they want "every scrap" of you until you are gone. So please write down your stories.

And if you are like me, with older generations still around to ask, let's commit this week to just ask.

What is something you wish you had asked someone before they were gone?

Write down one of your stories you want future generations to know.

A peek into my grandfather's mind

My grandfather passed away when I was in 4th grade. He was an insurance agent and a used car salesman, but fit none of the stereotypes. He was unfailingly honest and kind.

Years ago, while looking through some old papers I found a notebook where he recorded all his auto sales. Clearly listed in neat rows and excellent handwriting were the makes and models and years of each car as well as the purchaser and sales price.

About halfway down a page, in the middle of the notebook was an entry that said something like:

"1957 Ford Fairlane - red and white - coupe - automatic seats - for Cheryl"

A simple note, nestled in among all the rest, was a record of his own purchase of my mom's first car. They had buried the keys in the Christmas tree.

Another notebook detailed his fight to quit smoking. With dates and numbers and times of his habits, trying to reduce the number and frequency of his smoke breaks.

At the time, these records likely seemed inconsequential and unremarkable to him. But to me now, they are a priceless insight into the man I didn't ever get a chance to know. I'm so glad he kept them, and that I found them.

Write about a record you've found that gave you insight into someone's life.

What is a special gift you've given to someone?

Hot glue mistakes

Several years ago I was working on a craft project with my daughter. We were using hot glue. (Can you see where this is going?)

She was holding something for me, and I accidentally dripped hot glue on her finger. She screamed. I panicked and quickly swiped the glue off her finger. Which of course took with it a big chunk of her skin, making a bad situation much worse.

My instinct to quickly remove the painful situation from my children is one I have experienced repeatedly as they have grown older. I find myself wanting to jump in and remove any hurt or pain they might be experiencing.

But for the most part, I have refrained from rescuing them (except when it's my fault, like the Hot Glue Incident). I have found that as they sit with their pain, they learn to manage it. Learn from it. Resolve it, or at least find a way forward. I can be kind, attentive and compassionate. But that doesn't mean I solve everything for my kids. They need to learn that skill.

This is not just true for children, but it is true for me, too. Rather than wasting time wishing my frustrations and difficulties would just disappear–waiting for someone to rescue me–I should focus more on managing, learning from, and resolving painful situations myself.

Besides, if the Hot Glue Incident taught me anything, it's that rescue efforts sometimes make things worse.

Describe a time you wanted to rescue someone.
What happened? Would you do things differently?

Write about a challenge that helped you grow stronger because you faced it on your own.

Reaching for 11 when the limit is 10

I love being Aunt Diahan. It is one of my favorite roles.

Recently I was able to spend the day with my five nieces and nephews. We had a BLAST. We did a science project, played games, painted with face paint, ate pizza and cookies, crafted.

At one point we decided we needed music. My 7 year-old nephew had the following conversation with the smart speaker:

Nephew: Speaker, play (insert name of a song)
Speaker: Playing (insert name of song)
Nephew: Speaker, turn volume up to 100!
Me (thinking): Oh my....
Speaker: I'm sorry. I can only turn the volume to 10.
Nephew (with even more enthusiasm): Speaker, turn the volume to 11!

I laughed. But then I got to thinking about the demands that we place on ourselves and others. Sometimes we overestimate possibilities, like requesting a volume setting of 100 on a speaker. Taking a request from 100 to 11 makes 11 feel like it must be possible. But no matter its proximity, 11 is still impossible when the maximum is 10.

There are only so many hours in a day, so many ways you can stretch and maximize your time. I've decided I can do myself and everyone around me a favor when I respect the maximums and refuse to try to overshoot them. I hope you can set these limits too.

Write about a time you set unrealistic expectations for yourself or others.

How are you doing with the balance between contentment and stretching yourself?

Date

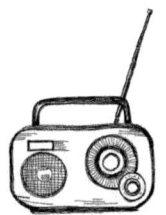

There's a cockroach on your back

Several years ago my husband and I walked out of a movie theater with a crowd of others. I removed my jacket as we left the cold air conditioning and emerged into the thick, humid south Florida evening.

Then I spotted something on the back of the woman in front of me. It was a huge cockroach, crawling up her back towards her shoulder.

I didn't even hesitate. My adrenaline surged and I whipped my jacket around and smacked it on her back, knocking the cockroach to the ground. She turned quickly, shocked. I sputtered how sorry I was but that there was a cockroach on her back. She thanked me, and we parted ways.

When was the last time you acted without thinking? Our first reactions aren't always in the best interest of ourselves or others, but they do tell us something about ourselves. It seems that we are acting from the core of who we are. Pure and unfiltered.

I am going to pay more attention to my gut reactions this week to see what I can learn about myself. I hope you will too. And if you're ever walking in front of me and a cockroach is crawling on you, don't worry. I've got your back.

Describe a time you acted on impulse. What did you learn about yourself?

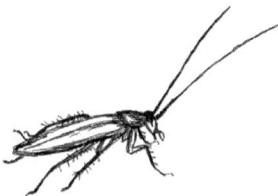

Driving in Canada with a poor sense of direction

Whenever I go to Canada, I forget that I am actually traveling to another country and things will be different. (Lovely, of course, but different.)

Also, my sense of direction is mediocre at best. So I fully rely on GPS directions to get me anywhere, even short distances. But when the GPS starts pointing me in the exact opposite direction of my destination, even I (with my poor sense of direction) start to feel like things are a little "off."

Last time I was in Canada, I did a bit of driving in the Toronto area. I found that If I wanted to go west along a certain route, I first had to go east, then flip a U-turn so I could start traveling in my desired direction. This was new to me.

This experience reminded me that sometimes the only way I can see to go seems to be the wrong way—if only because it feels uncomfortable and new and a little scary. But it could be that there's a U-turn coming up and I just don't see it. And, it seems that sometimes movement in any direction will just get my wheels moving. That momentum can propel me to my destination—even if I end up turning around a few times before I get there.

Direction and momentum—both important. So if you're stuck, just start moving, and you'll figure things out.

Write about a time you got lost, or went the wrong way.

How do you handle unexpected turns in life?

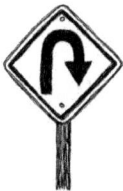

Reading my journal a year later

I keep a five-year journal. Each page has five spaces so I can look back and read what I wrote on the same day in prior years. It is usually entertaining and interesting. But for the one-year anniversary of my mother's passing, it was hard.

My mother was in hospice care, at home, with my sister and I caring for her, for 13 days before she passed. Here's what I wrote during those days:

23 May: "I got in my Uber at 3:30 AM...and was at my mom's (hospital) bedside by two...Mom just keeps repeating 'Home!' so that's the plan."

25 May: "A long night at the hospital. I slept in the reclining chair next to her bed. It felt like trying to sleep on an airplane with an infant. She would sleep for an hour and then I would wake up to her...trying to get out of bed to go home."

26 May: "So grateful Jared [my husband] and the kids are here. Eleanor [my daughter] sat by Nona's bed most of the day."

29 May: "All the nurses have talked about this transition period from life to death...I just can't quite actually convince myself that is where we are at with all of this."

2 June: "I haven't been keeping good records and every day is running into the next. Just more sitting and waiting."

4 June: "...She has not been at all responsive today."

6 June: "...When I woke up at 5:30 I stared at her chest like I have done so many times, waiting for her to take that big breath. But she didn't..."

As painful as these are to read, I am so grateful to have all of these details about what it was like those last days. Even after just a year I had forgotten some of the interactions, some of the visitors, and those precious moments. If you are not keeping a journal, it is time to start.

Have you ever revisited a painful memory? How had your perspective changed?

Write about a loss that changed you.

When I'm holding a box-knife

I bought a box of cereal the other day that had a big slash cut across the top. It made me laugh. I know exactly how that happened.

My first job was at a grocery store as a courtesy clerk. I was given my very own box-knife, just a simple blade in a sheath, that I would use to open boxes efficiently. I learned a technique for opening boxes so you don't damage the product inside. Whoever opened that pack of cereal boxes hadn't learned that lesson yet.

Which was why I was so impressed to receive a shipment of my own books. The ingenious packaging design made it impossible to damage the product inside, no matter how careless your knife skills. The company was protecting my books against my carelessness, even though any damage I might cause would not be their fault. Why would they bother?

I decided they cared about me as their customer so much that they were willing to take on a responsibility that wasn't actually theirs. Do I ever do that? Do I ever care so much about another person that I am willing to take steps to protect them from themselves, even when it is inconvenient for me and it might not even be my responsibility?

Certainly we do this with our children, but what about others? Should we even? This will be my thought to ponder this week.

What's a small, protective action you take to care for the people you love?

Write about a time someone protected you or your belongings.

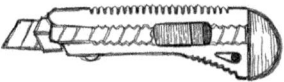

Tantrums and tactics: It wasn't really about me

My middle son had quite a temper as a kid. One day when he was about four or five, he was sent to his room. He started to yell at me from behind the door, banging on it occasionally for good measure.

"I hate you! And I hate dad! And I hate grandpa! And I hate Nona!" He listed everyone he could think of. Then you could tell he was running out of people and he said, "And I hate...WALMART!" I was glad he couldn't see me laughing.

But as he got older, his tactics got better for lashing out. He knew exactly what to say to me that would hurt the most. (Isn't that part of the trouble with letting people truly know us? The fear that we are handing them all the ammunition they need to really hurt us.)

I learned to recognize in those moments with my son that this was my sweet, kind, compassionate boy begging for love and understanding. He just felt so much, so deeply, that it was hard to contain sometimes.

I hope if you have a loved one in your life whose words seem to pierce you too effectively, that you will see their hurt, have compassion and try to help soothe their pain with your patience and understanding. And I hope that they, like my son, will soon grow out of the habit of lashing out at you. But if they don't, I hope that you will know the right thing to do next. Whatever it is.

How do you manage difficult emotions, and how do you help others manage theirs?

Describe a time someone's outburst hurt you. How did you handle it?

Date

What I learned from an ER doctor about triage

Recently an emergency room doctor described the triage process to me. When a person enters the ER, the intake doctor or nurse immediately assesses whether this person might die in the next five minutes. They run down a quick checklist. In those few minutes, they are in a state of super-high alert, ready to take quick action should they determine the patient needs it.

Once they know the person isn't in imminent danger, they can slow down and take their time to try to assess the problem and develop a plan.

When I get into a state of overwhelm, I tend to stay in that state of imminent danger. Sure, I have checklists, but I get stuck in that high-stimulation mode. I just bounce back and forth from one topic to the next, from one task to the next, often not accomplishing the most important things.

It would be like that ER doctor fixing someone's hangnail when another patient was bleeding out from a gaping wound in his abdomen.

Next time I'm in a frantic state, I'll try to channel the calm of the ER intake doctor or nurse, assess the situation, and take the next best steps to address any "gaping wound" situations–and know that eventually I'll get around to those less-critical hangnails, too.

Reflect on a time when you had to prioritize what mattered most.

What's something in your life that feels overwhelming right now? How can you triage it?

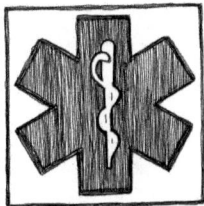

What lasts longer than balloons and flowers?

I love so many things about taking the train. One thing I love is that we get the backyard view that is mostly hidden from everyone else. We see unkempt backyards, dirty parking lots, and overgrown bushes. It's like looking at real life instead of whatever we pretty-up to present to the thoroughfares.

Recently I was taking the public train that picks up passengers a block from my house and runs all the way downtown. As I watched the scenery flash by, I saw a big trash heap piled with mylar balloons and rotting floral arrangements.

Wait. What was that? Then I remembered what zipped past just before the trash heap: a cemetery. These cast-off balloons and flowers were the remnants of the homage paid by loved ones at the graves of their departed.

This glimpse made me think how these gifts to our deceased loved ones have no permanence. It made me want to do something more lasting to honor those I love.

I believe we are accomplishing that when we build our family trees, share their stories and connect with other descendants. We are preserving something about them–their legacies–and that lasts so much longer than balloons and flowers.

Share a memory of a loved one, or a way you have honored their memory.

How do you hope to be remembered?

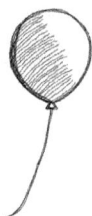

Strategies for sharing french fries

Early in my marriage, I realized that I needed to adjust how I ate french fries. At least, if I was sharing them with my husband.

See, my husband is what I now refer to as a compartmentalized eater. He eats one thing at a time. I am more of a grazer. I want a bite of this, then a little of that.

You can see the potential problem when a compartmentalist and a grazer try to share fries. If he eats his fries first, they may be mostly gone by the time I start grazing, even if he's not trying to eat more than his share. And of course he eats his fries first, because they get cold quickly. Which leaves me perpetually disadvantaged. And I like fries.

To get what I wanted (an equal share of fries), I needed to change a habit. I am sure I have changed lots of habits to accommodate new situations, but this is one I still have to do consciously. Whether he meant to or not, my husband helped me recognize this and adapt. It's not all bad. It means more of my fries are still warm! I know I could also ask him to change his habit, too. But I think I'll consider this one my secret service to him.

What adaptations have you made to navigate a situation more effectively? And has your partner or friend—just by being themselves—helped you to learn just a little bit more about yourself? That's always a good thing. At least as good as getting your share of (warm) fries.

Write about a relationship that caused you to change your habits.

What kinds of things do you like (and not like) to share?

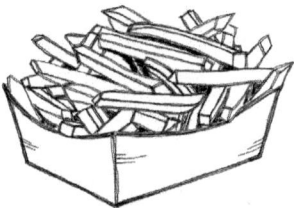

On claiming (or dropping) your baggage

I was in the baggage claim section of a large international airport when I noticed the sign: "Baggage Reclaim." In all the U.S. airports I have been to, the sign says "Baggage Claim."

Now, you might think that is just semantics. But it got me thinking. While "claim" always seemed like a perfectly perfect explanation of what was happening when we snatch up our luggage off the rotating belt, this new version of the word is so much better.

After all, you don't actually want to "claim" any old bag (nope, that black one is NOT yours, put it back on the belt). You want to "reclaim" your bag. Reclaim sounds personal. It feels like homecoming.

I started wondering what I may have lost that I should reclaim. What faith practices or relationship habits have I just let scroll by on the seemingly endlessly rotating belt of possible things to do that it is time to reach out and reclaim? After all, they are mine, or once were, and bringing them back into my life may be just the homecoming I need.

What about you? What will you reclaim this week?

What is something from your past you would like to reclaim?

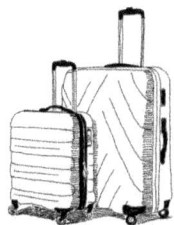

Is 80% good enough?

My brother-in-law emerged from the men's room at the concert hall, completely impressed. He practically waxed poetic about the fancy hardware for their sinks and urinals. He's a plumber.

So of course I started asking what makes one spigot better than another. I was most impressed by his trivia regarding the massive Allegiant Stadium in Las Vegas. Apparently the contracted plumber asked volunteers to come and stand at every toilet in the stadium—and flush at the same time. The plumber wanted to be sure every single toilet in the entire stadium could flush simultaneously without mishap. They can, by the way.

It got me thinking about how that plumber wanted to be prepared for an extremely unlikely event. Wouldn't it have been good enough to design a system that would handle 80% capacity simultaneous flushing?

I am honestly not sure where I fall on that whole efficiency vs perfection scale on most days. Most of the time I say I am good with the 80%, but then my actions often belie that declaration. I strive for perfection even when I say I know that 80% is enough. Because most of the time, I think it is.

So this week I am going to be grateful, and even excited, about 80%, knowing that the 20% I am giving up will be much better spent toward a different project's 80%. What about you?

What does 'good enough' mean to you in different areas of your life?

Think of a time when you aimed for perfection. What happened?

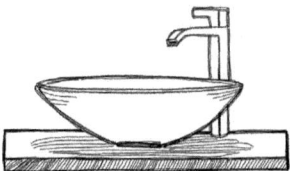

Patriotism, war machines, and the value of every life

I had the opportunity to attend an air show with my husband and my father, who is a U.S. Air Force veteran. It was hot, with temperatures near 100° F.

Unlike my dad, who has personal experiences to share from his years as an Explosives Ordnance Demolition Airman, and my husband (who I swear knows the names and specs of every aircraft), I know nothing about planes, and I thought I didn't have much interest.

I was wrong. It was fascinating. Impressive. Patriotic.

And then came a reenactment of the attack on Pearl Harbor. The chaos, the noise, the panic were all evident. I gained a much better appreciation for what military service men and women can face. What anyone faces when war rains down on them.

And then came the B2 bomber. Of course I have heard of it, but I didn't really understand its presence and power until it went from a speck in the north sky to a massive, coal black, SILENT wing overhead. Wow. Just WOW. I had so many questions. How does it fly? How does it do so silently? And most importantly, why did we create something that–when loaded with its deadly cargo–can so effectively snuff out so much human life so quickly?

While I understand the need for war at times, I empathize with those whose lives are torn apart on all sides of a conflict. Conflict is messy, confusing, and so difficult to fully grasp all the nuances of. But the value of a human life will always be the same in every battle, in every conflict, on every front. We are none of us more valuable than the other.

So while my brain marvels at this feat of engineering that is the flying machine, my heart hurts for all the lives it can affect. And I will do my best, in my own small sphere, to show how much I value each individual person.

Write about a time your life was touched by violence or war. What do you want to say about it?

What does patriotism mean to you, and how do you express it?

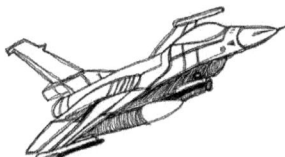

When you already have part of the solution

I recently looked over my husband's shoulder while he was working a crossword puzzle. My eyes scanned the puzzle and found a 6-letter word he had completed ACROSS that subsequently gave the first letters for all of those DOWN clues. So my eyes flicked over to the DOWN clues and I easily found an answer.

When I tried to point it out, my husband was, shall we say, less-than-pleased? No, that's not quite strong enough. Incredulous. It turns out that it wasn't the fact that I was "helping," but rather my methodology that he found so offensive. Apparently it is "more fun" to go through all the ACROSS clues first before you move to the DOWN.

As far as I'm concerned, that is just too much work! Why not solve a crossword puzzle by starting with one word and then just building out from that word, using your current letters to answer future clues? I can't even imagine starting over with no letters to go on almost every time you are looking at an ACROSS clue.

No matter how you crossword, I hope you are figuring out your current life challenges by building on your current knowledge and successes. I hope you don't feel like you are consistently starting over from scratch.

In my experience, there is always something that you have already learned that if you build on it, will help you through the next thing you're facing.

Reflect on a challenge where you built on past knowledge to find a solution.

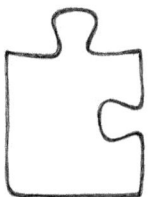

"That's not really my job"

I spoke at an in-person conference earlier this year. One of my favorite things to do.

However, I can be picky about the setup of my room. This room was a traditional hotel ballroom, with a big screen in front and a slightly elevated stage with a podium and a long table for panel discussions. But I like to have an empty stage so I can walk around.

In my first assigned room, I asked the man who was in charge of audio if it was OK to move the table off the stage. He said, "Sure, why not?" and started towards the stage to help me move it.

In the second room, to a different audio man, I made the same suggestion. He looked at the table as if it was some foreign object, and said with disdain, "That's not really my job." Me being me, I went to move it myself. Reluctantly, he started helping.

As I reflected on how differently those two men behaved in the very same situation, I started to wonder if I ever leave someone without the help they need simply because I don't consider it my job to help them.

Of course, sometimes people need more than I can give. Or something I don't know how to give. But moving a table? That's such a simple need. A lot of times, people just need something simple from me, too.

Is it ever NOT my job to see someone in need and NOT help in some way? Even if an encouraging smile is all I can offer? Next time I'm tempted to brush off a request with "That's not really my job," I hope I stop and consider what I CAN do. And that whatever I can or can't do, I'm kind about it.

Reflect on a situation where someone helped you when they didn't have to.

How do you define your responsibilities for helping others?
Has that changed over time?

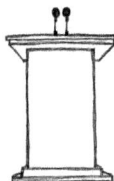

A policy that's not just for light switches

"Turn off the juice when not in use."

The phrase, in red lettering on a white sticker, was stuck to every light switch in my house growing up. My dad worked for the public utilities company, and paid attention to energy conservation.

I find myself repeating that phrase over and over every morning after everyone has left for school or work and I am wandering around the house turning off all the lights.

Lately I have been thinking about how I need to apply this phrase to my own self. I love my job and there is so much to do so I often eat lunch at my desk, and end up on the computer at night to just do a few more things before bed. But I know it makes a difference when I "turn off the juice" periodically throughout the day. Walk the dog. Talk to my family. Be still.

If you are at all like me, here is the reminder for both of us, whether it's the energy in your house or in your body: Turn off the juice when not in use. And don't be in use all the time!

Write about a time when stillness or "turning off" was the best thing for you.

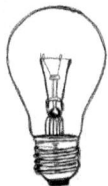

The bases are loaded—and you're pitching

The other night, my husband and I watched the minor league Salt Lake Bees play. When the opposing team switched out their pitcher in the middle of the inning, I thought about the weight of what he inherited from the previous pitcher: bases loaded, one out, already down by several runs.

Interestingly, this pitcher who was thrown into the middle of this inning was not held accountable for any runners who were already on base when he started. Even if he lobs in a big fat strike that gets hit into the next county in a grand slam home run, he was only responsible for the run scored by the hitter, not the other three that were still on base. Those were counted against his predecessor.

It made me think of how unevenly life can be distributed among us. How for some, as soon as they are born, the deck is stacked against them.

The choices and mistakes of those around us certainly impact our experience, even though we are not accountable for their choices. But at some point, the choices we make are our own.

For me, just understanding the field I have inherited—what was already put into play before I came on the field, so to speak—helps me to better focus on my responsibility for the actions that are my own.

I hope you can do the same.

What's a challenge or responsibility you inherited?

What life lesson have you learned from sports?

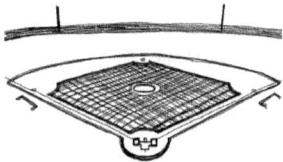

Biscoff butter and being who you are

Aebleskivers are Swedish filled pancakes. I was introduced to them by my Australian neighbor. You have to use a special pan, and it takes at least an hour to make the entire batch, six at a time.

The very best filling to use is Biscoff butter. Have you tried this stuff?! It is heaven in a jar. It is made from those fancy Biscoff cookies that I used to only find on an airplane. Now (sometimes) I find the Biscoff butter on store shelves next to the peanut butter.

Recently my daughter suggested that "we" make aebleskivers. So I headed to the store. But the Biscoff butter was not with the peanut butter or by the cookies. A helpful sales person said I would find it in the bakery, on a little wire shelf by the doughnuts. I must have looked at her strangely, as she went on to explain that Biscoff, the company, wanted to send a clear message: they weren't just some regular kind of cookie or cookie butter. They were a bakery item.

As I left the store I thought how silly it was that this cookie butter was putting on airs. It was trying to be something it wasn't, and in the process, it was lost in the store.

I do that sometimes. I try to be someone I am not, and get lost in the process. This week I am going to be confident in who I am instead of trying to be someone I am not. Want to join me?

And if you're looking for the Biscoff butter (because of course you are now), it may be in the bakery aisle. You're welcome.

Reflect on a time you embraced your true self--or tried to be someone you're not.

How do you stay true to yourself in situations where you might feel pressured to change?

Winning at cards

King's Corner is one of my favorite card games. Likely because I used to play it with my grandma in the mornings before she would walk me to my elementary school. I still play it often with my family and my dad.

For those of you unfamiliar with the game, you have four spaces on the playing board where you can play cards in descending order from king to ace, alternating them black and red, creating individual "runs." Often you can move a run from one space to another, leaving an open space where you can play any card from your hand.

Everyone who plays with me knows how my pet peeve is when someone plays an ace in an open spot. Because nothing comes after the ace, that play effectively seals that spot, limiting the playing options for everyone in the game.

I see it as a purely selfish move: trying to offload a relatively useless card from their hand onto the rest of us. My policy is to always play something that can be built on, trusting that if I do, that will open up opportunities for myself later to play all the cards in my hand. My strategy usually works, as I win more than I lose.

This principle has me reflecting on other times in my life when I selfishly put forth my own agenda, effectively shutting down the ideas or opinions of others. I think I am just being strategic or even clever, but that is rarely the case. By not allowing others to build or grow my ideas, those ideas effectively stagnate, and block progress. Not a good strategy. This week, I am not going to play my aces, but maybe a nice eight of hearts, and let's see what we can build on that, shall we?

What does one of your game-playing strategies say about you?

What's a 'selfish move' you've made, and how would you handle it differently now?

On leaving the garbage behind you

One of the most surprising and beneficial things about living in Broward County, Florida was the garbage collection service. You could put literally anything on the curb for pickup.

This is not the case in Centralia, Washington, where I grew up. In fact, over the last several visits to see my parents, I have made consistent trips to the dump. I began to really appreciate the ingenious system they use to charge you for whatever you have to get rid of.

You pull up to the little window where your entire vehicle is weighed, and you are handed a card that reports the weight of your load going in. Then after you unload, you come back to the other side of that building, hand them your card, and you are weighed again.

A simple calculation has you paying per pound for the difference in weight. No questions or detailed inventory. No judgment about what you were throwing away. Just straightforward, unbiased assessment of before and after.

This process feels so good. I always feel like I myself am personally lighter as we drive away.

All of us are carrying some kind of weight on our shoulders. This week--today even-- I hope you look around for your safe place or person or God where you can dump your burdens, without judgment, and move forward without them.

Reflect on a time when you felt lighter after releasing something from your life.

Is there a burden you'd like to let go of?

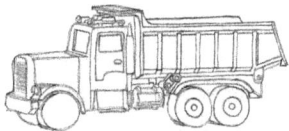

We can slow down time (sort of)

When was the last time you had a truly new experience? On a podcast a while ago, I heard that when we have a new experience, it feels like time slows way down.

That's probably about to happen for my daughter. I just dropped her off at a two-week theater camp: a totally new experience for her. I am so proud of her for going so far outside of her comfort zone, risking loneliness and vulnerability.

She is brave, friendly and resilient. But even so, for my daughter, the next two weeks will go by so slowly (which may be difficult, if she gets homesick) because she is having so many new experiences.

For me, time will speed by while she is gone. I want to plan something new so I won't feel like the time is passing too quickly. According to internet wisdom, there are lots of things I can try. I can seek new people or experiences, like my daughter is. I can learn something new and challenging, or dive deeply into solving a complicated problem. (Thank you, genetic genealogy, for always offering me a chance to slow down time!)

But I may not even have to work that hard to slow down time. I can pay more attention to the experiences I'm already living, looking for what's unique or special about them. I can even rearrange my furniture so things feel new. Maybe I'll rearrange my daughter's furniture instead, so she can keep having new experiences when she gets back home!

I hope your week passes at just the right pace for you–and that if time seems to be passing you by, you'll find lovely ways to slow it down.

Reflect on a new experience that made time feel slower.

What small changes can you make to savor the present moment more?

Scuba diving wasn't for me

As I slowly and helplessly floated back to the surface, I watched my scuba diving class swim along the reef below and away from me. My head broke the surface of the ocean, and I really started to panic.

I was supposed to love this. I needed to love this. My husband was completely passionate about this hobby. I'd been reading and practicing-diving for weeks so we could have this shared connection. In my head, I was already planning for many years of exotic, romantic scuba diving vacations.

I managed to take a deep breath and push the little button that released air from my gear. I slid back down to the seafloor and rejoined my class. Eventually I got my certification and did some dives with my husband. I loved the time with him, and experiencing the colors, serenity and beauty of life along the reef.

But I didn't love all the things. I discovered I get seasick fairly easily, even under the water. I always feel a little bit claustrophobic while diving, and it takes concentrated effort to relax about going under the water.

My biggest takeaway? We don't have to love the same things in the same way. He could be passionate about scuba diving, and I didn't have to be. He could go all the time, and I could go every so often. And that's ok.

Maybe you've already learned this about relationships. I hope you enjoy your most important friendships this week, whether you're hanging out together or each pursuing your own thing. I...will not be scuba diving. But we do have plans for a bike ride.

Reflect on a time when you tried something new for the sake of a relationship.

Sent to the principal's office

I was a bit of a smarty-pants in school. (Maybe this doesn't surprise you.) Today I'm going to tell you about a moment where I wasn't so smart, after all.

It was 6th grade. I had a teacher who was new to our small-town school district. She was somewhat surly and unimpressive. Then one day, I noticed something different when I walked into her classroom. There were maps and charts up everywhere, and she had turned into a picture of charm and kindness. Wondering at this change, I spotted our principal sitting in the corner.

I was on very friendly terms with my principal, as all smarty-pants kids are wont to be. I was somewhat disgusted by this show that my teacher was putting on for her superior, and I was determined to put her in her place. So when she called on me to read aloud, (undoubtedly believing she could trust me to show her in a good light), I completely over-dramatized the reading, drawing snickers from my classmates but to the utter embarrassment of my teacher.

I smugly went through the day, feeling I had won. But punishment came the next day in the form of detention (which I had never received in my 11 years). I was incensed. I marched myself right up to the principal's office, determined to tattle on my cruel teacher. As fate would have it, he was out of the office for the day.

Thankfully. Now I can see that my poor teacher was struggling to stay afloat in an unfamiliar place with unfamiliar people. Instead of trying to be kind or understanding, I tried to show her up.

I hope, next time you see someone struggling, you'll be kind instead of a smarty-pants. I'll try, too. It is worth the effort.

Write about a time when you gave an authority figure a hard time.

In what situations could you offer more grace and kindness?

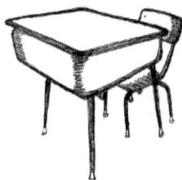

No MVP award for me—but this was better

When I was a young teenager, I went to NBC basketball camp in Eastern Washington. I loved the cabins and the cafeteria food and the girls I met. I love playing basketball. Wednesdays were the dreaded defense day where you spent nearly the entire day in a wall-sit, or in a defensive position (which is basically a wall sit without the wall). It was HARD. But I survived.

On the last day of camp they gathered all 300 or so of us into one big auditorium for a closing ceremony. Tournament winners were given trophies. Those who had achieved the highest scores in free-throws, rebounds, and three point shots were also awarded. I didn't earn any of those. I was a decent player, but nothing to write home about.

We left just before the ceremony to get me to a fastpitch softball tournament. But I learned later that there was an unexpected award given: for the one girl in the entire camp who was the most inspirational.

It was me.

And that honor meant more to me than any other award could. I would never be the best basketball player, but I could help make others better.

"Most inspirational" is a role anyone can play at a crucial moment for someone they love. Be there. Care. And be willing to do hard things when the stakes are high.

Hopefully you won't have to wall-sit.

Reflect on a moment when you inspired others, or someone inspired you.

Think of a situation now where you would like to inspire someone more.

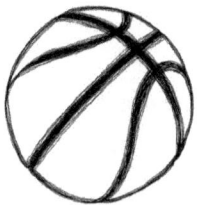

Are you this passionate about what you do?

Hair mussed, my son emerged from the back of the dentist's office to join my other two children, with similarly disheveled hair, in the lobby. He gave me the classic teenage eye-roll as I headed toward the back office (with much more enthusiasm than they did).

The woman behind the desk greeted me with a wide smile and said with beautifully accented English, "Hello Mrs. Southard! How are you? I love that yellow purse!"

I sat in the chair across from her desk and the gushing began: how darling my kids were, how much they had grown, etc. But as she tilted the computer monitor towards me, her entire demeanor changed. Accolades were replaced with true pain (I'm not exaggerating) as she gestured at the black and white images and detailed the failings of my children's oral hygiene.

Dr. Portilla may be the thing I miss very most about moving away from Florida. It's not just that she was an excellent pediatric dentist. It's because she is just so passionate about teeth–specifically, the teeth of MY children. She explained everything to me as if we shared the same interest and training, and because she really wanted me to catch this vision of dental care that she saw so clearly.

I want to be like her. I want every person I interact with to feel my genuine care for them and my commitment to helping them catch a vision of what is possible with their DNA. And I hope you, in turn, have someone who inspires YOU to be the most passionate advocate for what you care about most.

Reflect on a time when you were inspired by someone's dedication to their craft.

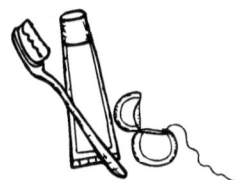

How butter revealed my core value

A couple weeks ago I was in a hurry to soften butter to make cobbler, so I threw the butter in the microwave for a few seconds. I opened the microwave to a melted mess. See, I had put the butter in without a dish. Just in its wrapper. Which was now swimming in a buttery puddle.

My husband, who would never commit such a kitchen atrocity, shook his head knowingly at me, then looked at my son and said, "One of mom's core values is to not use too many dishes."

It's true. Even in the age of dishwashers, I am always trying to minimize the dirty dishes, often to my detriment, as you see.

Long after I cleaned up my mess and we had eaten the cobbler, I was thinking of how powerful it is to understand the core values of another person. Even though my husband and I don't hold the same view about dish use, he was kind because he understands what motivates me. This has inspired me to try to more fully understand the core values of those around me, and once identified, to not judge them or belittle them. Instead, I can just recognize and love them for who they are right now. This helps especially with teenagers, whose core values are way out of alignment with my own.

I hope you will have a chance this week to recognize core values in yourself or others, and allow that awareness to make things a little better for everyone.

What are your core values, and how do they shape your daily decisions?

Share a time when your core values were clearly different from someone else's. What happened?

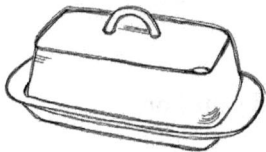

What "you do you" really means

"You do you." How many times have you heard that in the last week? I feel like I hear it all the time. At the outset, it seems like we shouldn't argue with this premise. Aren't we always supposed to be true to ourselves?

Yes, AND...I think "You do you" is an incomplete thought that implies that everyone can just go their own way. Which isn't realistic or even desirable. Inevitably, we have to cross paths with others. We *want* to cross paths.

I think it should be, "You do you so we can be the best us." Our own unique abilities are meant to complement and accent the unique abilities of another. In a country, in a community, and certainly in a family or friendship. Sometimes you have to "do you" *in a way that fits with another person or group.*

In any given group scenario, you might have to sacrifice the volume or genre of your music or your choice of activity for a Friday night so that the "us" part of your group can be together.

This week as you "do you," I invite you to consider how you adapt your usual "you" for those around you. Do you invite a better "us" (whatever that "us" is for you)? Do you recognize and appreciate when others adapt for you, maybe meet you halfway?

I'm going to try to open my own door a little wider, to show people I love that I want to be a better "us," and notice when they do the same.

Write about a relationship you'd like to improve.

Write about a time when giving someone more space strengthened your bond.

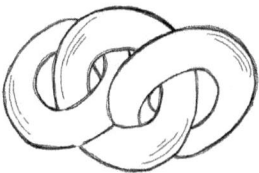

What we think others are thinking

A few Sundays ago I put my unwashed hair up in a high ponytail, put on a newish modern cut sweater shirt thingy and a plain blue skirt. Looking at myself in the mirror I thought, "Good enough," and I went downstairs.

My husband was in the kitchen. When I came in, he looked at me for a long moment. I thought I could hear him thinking: "Mmm, interesting shirt–and meh on the third-day hair."

Later that afternoon, as we were sitting at the table with our daughter playing cards, she said she'd thought her dad was staring her down from the front of the church when she walked in with me. Then she realized he was looking at me.
"Really?" I asked.

My husband then said, "Yes, I just couldn't stop looking at you. I love it when you wear your hair in a ponytail."

I realized what I had imagined he was thinking earlier that morning couldn't have been further from the truth. What I heard in my own head were my own insecurities about myself, not his actual criticism of me. I do that too often. I let my own negative thoughts masquerade as the unspoken thoughts of others.

I am going to try to just listen to what is actually being said to me, instead of conjuring unkind thoughts in my head and blaming them on others. I hope you will too.

Reflect on a time when you allowed your insecurities to cloud a situation.

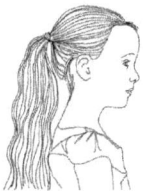

Calling home with a lost phone

I was milling about in a high school gymnasium after a volleyball game, waiting for my son. Teenagers and parents stood around in small groups, chatting. Then a boy noticed an abandoned phone on the bleachers and held it in the air. "Did someone forget their phone?"

No one claimed it. A girl standing next to him took the phone and, pressing the button on the side of it, said, "Call Mom."

Wasn't that the most clever idea?!

I love how "calling mom" on any one phone will get you a very specific person, even though the name applies to millions of people. There may be millions of moms out there, but only one is yours. (Except for those blessed families that have a bonus mom, of course!)

As for the lost phone? As the girl was chatting with "mom" about her son's lost phone, he showed up and claimed it. A bit embarrassed that some random strange girl had been chatting with his mom, but at least he got his phone back.

Reflect on a memory or feeling about your mother or father.

Who would others call to find you?

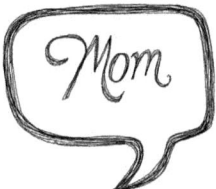

Mom

When approaching a yellow light

Have you ever marveled at the genius of the yellow signal in a traffic light? While it is jokingly referred to as the "go faster" signal where I live, its true purpose is to gently transition you from motion to stillness.

I am in the midst of one of these transition times right now.

Both my sons are off making their own way in the world. My 16 year-old daughter–the only child at home–is rarely in the house. She's at school, work, friends, and marching band.

My husband and I find ourselves in a big, empty house.

My coping mechanism is to just stay busy, to stay in motion to not feel the loss of the boys I miss so much.

The other day I was feeling a bit melancholy about this and my husband said something profound: "When all of the stress and worry fades, this is going to be really fun."

At that moment, I thought of the yellow light. This is a transition time that I have been trying to rush through. Instead perhaps I should slow down, and even stop, and appreciate that this transition time deserves its moment.

Write about a time of transition in your life. How did you manage it?

Reflect on a time you wish you would have slowed down.

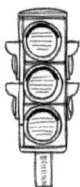

Speaking the language of teenagers

I absolutely love teenagers. But it must be very difficult to be a teacher of teenagers these days. In any day and age it was probably tricky. Now you have to contend with more than just hormones and awkwardness, like smart phones and Netflix.

My daughter's 9th grade Environmental Science teacher is doing an exceptional job. One small thing she does is take standard material and make it relevant for her 14 and 15 year old audience. For example, on a reading guide the other day I spotted:

"In 1989 Taylor Swift was born and it was also the year of the Exxon Valdez oil spill that..." Don't you love it? She added just a simple hook at the beginning of the line to make the material relevant to her audience.

Connecting with teens means I have to learn to speak their language. To do that, I actually need to talk to them more. I hope you have a teenager in your life. I challenge you to just talk to them more. They need you. They need your knowledge and experience and reassurance that life really does go on, in spite of its challenges. They need to know we are cheering them on.

Write a memory about being a teenager.

How do you connect with younger generations?

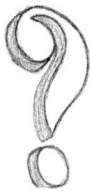

Furniture shopping compromises

A while ago, I was at a big homegoods store. I needed a picture frame, and I knew exactly where it was. But I still wandered slowly though the other sections of the store.

I started observing the couples who were also shopping. There was very specific body language and hand gestures. They would lean their heads together slightly as they observed a couch or coffee table. They would mime the dimensions of the room and show with their hands where they saw this fitting in their shared space.

There was quite a bit of back and forth as one partner would argue for their choice, and the other would try to better explain their position. But the goal was the same: co-creating a space that meant something to both of them.

I love all the hope and possibility of moments like that, when people work together toward their common goal. When, with a friend or loved one or partner or colleague, you envision something different or better for your shared space. I love to see how people with different ideas can ultimately settle on something that works for them both. Compromises have to be made, accommodations even for a color or fabric that the other feels strongly about.

I am going to try to appreciate the compromises my people have made for me. I'm going to make sure I tell them that this week.

Reflect on a compromise you've made to share space with someone else.

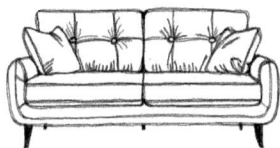

Just ask

I love my birthday. It is my favorite holiday.

My husband and I have this unspoken rule: No birthday presents. We value experiences over things, so we would often plan something fun together or as a family, and we would certainly always go out to dinner and have some yummy dessert.

But I found myself disappointed, year after year. I kept hoping my fabulous husband would surprise me with a gift. One year, we were actually in Norway over my birthday. (I was speaking at the first MyHeritage LIVE event, and so it made a nice excuse for him to join me on a getaway.) On the morning of my birthday I was getting ready to speak, and my husband kissed me goodbye and wished me a happy birthday. That's it. No gift.

"What's wrong with me?" I thought. I am in Norway on vacation with my favorite person!! What more did I want for my birthday?!

So the next year I decided to say something. I just told my husband that for whatever irrational reason, I required a gift on my birthday. It did not need to be expensive, just something I did not pick out myself. No more expecting him to read my mind, no more feeling guilty for wanting something.

And guess what? He came through (of course he did!). Why did I wait so long?

If there is something you need, that you just haven't had the courage to ask for, ask for it today. And whenever your next birthday is, I hope it's a happy one.

What is something you've been wanting to ask for but haven't yet?

Write about a gift you've given or received.

Who is your silly song and dance person?

My 3rd grade teacher was Mrs. Winningham. At the end of the school day she would often play a song, and we would sing and dance. That's when I learned the 50 states song (ask me to sing it next time you see me; I still love it).

In the fall, as Halloween approached, we would sing the song, "Witches' Brew." The verses listed all kinds of things we were adding to our brew, like fingernails and rotten eggs, and then the chorus said, "Stir them in my witches' brew, I got magic, alakazamakazoo."

I can picture my teacher, up in the front of the room singing this song. She has a big smile on her face. Her left arm circles out from her body, in cauldron shape, while her right arm holds her pretend spoon and turns in big wide circles. She is doing a little dance with her feet in time with the music.

Why is that such a crisp memory after all these years? The song is catchy, yes, but that's not it. I think it is the way she was looking at me and my classmates. I think I could feel how much she loved me. I think the combination of the music and the fun feeling in the room just helped her to show even more of how she felt.

I hope you have someone you love with whom you can sing a silly song or have a bit of fun. In fact, why don't you go do it? I think it will help them feel how much you care.

How do you incorporate fun and whimsy into your relationships?

Reflect on a time when you connected with others through fun traditions.

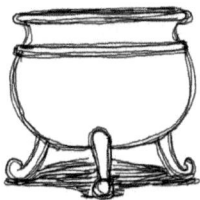

What do you hope they'll remember about you?

My husband and I never miss our date night. Our favorite thing to do is just go out to eat and talk.

One night was particularly hectic, with different kids needing to be dropped off in different locations on opposite sides of town. After meeting for dinner at a restaurant, we stood in the parking lot, discussing mundane, married-for-a-long-time kind of things, like grocery lists and carpool schedules. I stood on the curb, so although he is much taller, we were nearly eye to eye. Then we parted ways to our separate cars and continued our busy evening.

Afterward, my husband called to say that someone had been watching us talk on the curb. As he walked past her, she said to him, "You should have kissed her!"

I love how a stranger mistook two old married people for a couple in the blush of new love, too nervous to kiss goodbye. I love that I still feel that flutter of excitement when I see him. I love that we are still in love, even after 20 years together.

I am writing this story down so my grandchildren and great grandchildren will know that we were more than two names in their family tree. We had a story. A love story.

What do you want future generations to know about you? Write it down.

What's a story you would like your family to remember about you?

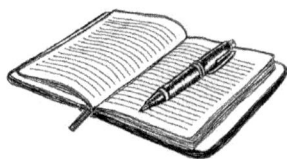

I'm not judging. I'm just curious. Right?

"The past is a foreign country. They do things differently there." - L.P. Hartley

I could probably write an entire essay–hey, maybe even a book–about all the thoughts this quote makes me think. Today it makes me think about how I want to give my ancestors space to have lived only in their own time and place, and not impose my modern-day views or values on the choices they made.

That tendency to judge the people of the past based on the views of the present is what genealogists call "presentism." I don't want to JUDGE my ancestors. I just want to be curious about them.

I want to learn more about their worldview and their culture and their circumstances so I can better understand their story as they would have told it. Not their story the way I would tell it.

I would want them to do the same for me. After all, I wander around nearly every day in men's trousers with my ankles scandalously uncovered, right? (Or at least, that's what some of my ancestors would think if they chose to judge me according to their own values.) That wouldn't be fair, would it? So I'll try to extend them the same courtesy.

I do wish I could tell the women just how comfortable these trouser things are, though.

Write a story about an ancestor who lived differently than you.

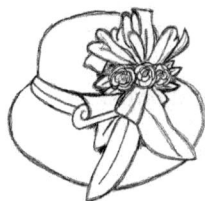

Memorable moments and inflatable sticks

I love to play games. Board games, card games, it doesn't matter. I am grateful that my husband and kids like to play as well. Bored with playing the same games, recently we bought some new ones.

One is called Poetry for Neanderthals. You have to get your team to guess the word or words on your card but you can only give your clues in one-syllable words. The fun part–for teenagers and adults alike–is that it comes with an inflatable stick. So if you say a word that is more than one syllable, someone on the other team gets to beat you with the stick.

Here's how it played out at my house: My daughter was trying to get me to guess "duck" and she started to say the word "yellow." But halfway through, she realized that "yellow" is two syllables, so she said "yell" [big pause] then "oh." Then she proceeded to get struck on the head by her brother with the inflatable stick.

It was actually really funny.

We have noticed how much you can say, even using simple words. But also how frustrating it is when you can't use the words you need.

If you have a group of friends or family that need some entertainment (or you have someone you would like to beat with an inflatable, non-injury-causing stick), I highly recommend this game. It helps make memorable moments. And don't we all need more of those?

Write about a memorable, fun time you've enjoyed with friends or loved ones.

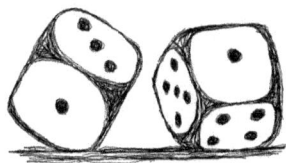

Ice makes me grateful

I try to drink as much water as I can every day. There is something almost Pavlovian about getting in the car that makes me immediately thirsty, so I always bring water with me. Icy cold water.

That requires plenty of ice, and sometimes flavoring. I am currently obsessed with this green fruity flavor. When flavored, the ice-to-water ratio needs to heavily favor the ice, so the flavor is really strong.

So it's definitely inconvenient that our in-the-fridge ice maker randomly turns off and stops producing ice. The thing is, no one seems to realize this until we are completely out of ice. This has been happening often lately.

Every time I open the freezer and see a full tray of ice, I feel a palatable relief. I feel actual, real, true gratitude that there is so much ice that I can have as much as I want to. I know, it's a little thing, a simple pleasure. And yet I am grateful for it.

I hope that you are feeling all the gratitude "feels" this week, even for simple pleasures.

What simple pleasure are you grateful for today?

Write about an inconvenience that made you appreciate something even more.

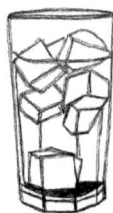

A simple tree or full-blown holiday decor?

I fully intended to be one of those people who decorate for every holiday. With lights and wreaths and figurines and even different throw pillows for the couch. I love a festive home!

Much to my dismay, I am not that person. I don't want to spend money on holiday decorations or take time to shop for them. I don't want the bother of putting things up, taking them down, and storing all those things.

So because I love the way a decorated home looks, but I am obviously not willing to do the work to make it happen, I love the power and simplicity of the Christmas tree. It has so much natural beauty, and it doesn't have to be perfectly decorated to brighten the entire room with the Christmas spirit. I find myself sitting in my living room, just looking at my tree. And it's enough.

At Christmas time, perhaps more than any other time, no one should feel less-than. It can be hard to feel like you have done enough or if you ARE enough.

So I just wanted to take the chance to tell you. You are enough.

Reflect on a time when you felt "enough" without doing more.

Write about a memory of holiday decorations or celebrations.

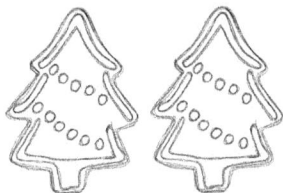

Here's to the courtesy clerks at checkout

When I was a teenager, I was a courtesy clerk ("bagger") at a locally-owned grocery store. I simultaneously loved and hated holiday cooking season.

I loved watching all the shoppers with their huge long lists, and the similarities and differences in everyone's carts. Turkey, potatoes, stuffing, and rolls were in nearly everyone's cart. Some bought nuts with their sweet potatoes, and some marshmallows. Some bought corn with cream and others green beans with onions. Some apple pie, some pumpkin pie.

Shoppers were always full of anticipatory energy. (Not always positive energy, mind you, but it was mostly positive.) Everyone was looking forward to gatherings and games and good food. Most were feeling thankful and generous: that came through in their interactions with me and others.

But who was it that had to bag all those groceries into perfectly proportioned bags (yes, we were trained and tested on how to make the perfectly balanced bag of groceries)? Who had to lug those 25 lb turkeys and multitude of other groceries out to their car?

It was me. And it was usually raining; after all, I lived in Washington state.

So among the lists you have of things to be thankful for this year, perhaps you could add your lowly courtesy clerk to the list? That is, unless you shop where you have to bag your own groceries, in which case, I know you feel my pain.

What was something you learned from your first job?

Reflect on a time when you were grateful for someone who made your day easier.

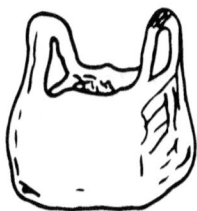

Filling the holiday cup

I spent several holiday seasons bagging groceries. This was back in the mid to late nineties and my sheltered, middle-class self learned some hard lessons about the world.

Back then, if you used government assistance to purchase food, there wasn't a discreet credit card system. You had to actually rip food stamps or WIC checks out of a booklet.

Around the holiday seasons, the grocery orders got bigger and heavier and those booklets got lighter and lighter. Moms and dads were trying to put food on the table and buy a little extra candy for those stockings. On more than one occasion, I saw people who didn't have enough left in their booklets to pay for the groceries in their cart. They were forced to put things back. It was heart wrenching.

I often think back to that time as I throw items into my grocery cart. This year I find myself in a place of relative abundance. If you are like me, I hope you will find a way to give back in the form of your money or your food. If you find yourself a little thin this year, I hope that you will find what you need, and I also invite you to give your time. So many food banks and shelters need our help.

Let's all work together to fill more people's holiday cups this holiday season.

What do you have in abundance to share? How can you share more of it?

Write about a time when you filled a need, or someone filled yours.

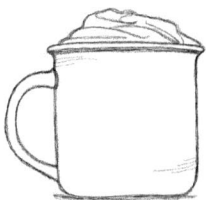

"Preserve your memories, keep them well, what you forget can never retell." - Louisa May Alcott

www.ingramcontent.com/pod-product-compliance
Lightning Source LLC
Chambersburg PA
CBHW081147020426
42333CB00021B/2690